TEA FOR DIABETES

"A Comprehensive Guide to Managing Blood Sugar"

By

Linda a. Ivey

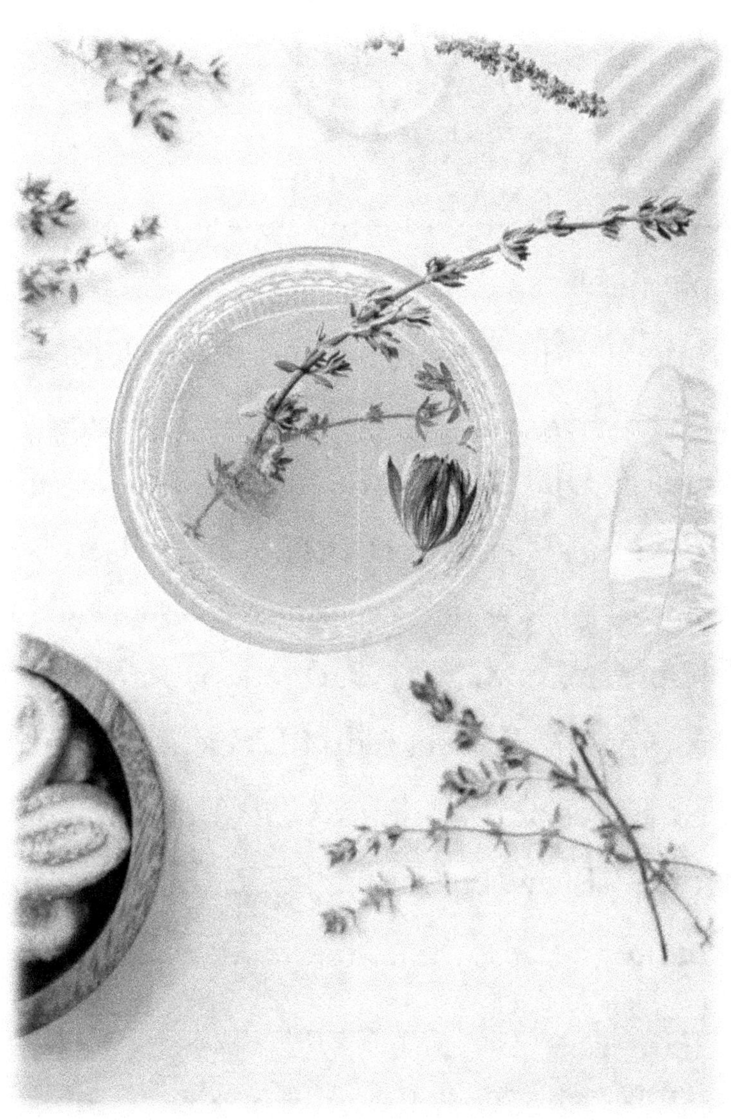

Table of Contents

Introduction 4

Chapter 1 8

Understanding Diabetes and the Role of Tea 8

What is Diabetes? 8

How Does Tea Affect Blood Sugar Levels? 11

Chapter 2...24

Brewing the Perfect Cup of Tea 24

Tea Types and Varieties 24

How to Brew Tea.................................32

Chapter 3...40

Black Tea Recipes.................................40

Chapter 4...58

Green Tea Recipes 58

Chapter 5 69

White Tea Recipes...............................69

Chapter 6 79

Herbal Tea Recipes 79

Chapter 7 91

Fruit Tea Recipes 91

Chapter 8 104

Iced Tea Recipes.......................104

Conclusion 116

Glossary terms.........................119

Index 127

Introduction

Diabetes is a disorder that develops when your body is unable to produce enough insulin or utilize it effectively. A substance called insulin regulates the body's glucose levels. When blood glucose levels are too high, it can result in various problems, including cardiovascular disease, nerve damage, kidney damage, and eye damage. While including tea in your routine might provide additional benefits, the three main components of diabetic management are medication, a healthy diet, and regular exercise. Polyphenols are plant compounds found in tea that have the ability to strengthen cells and reduce inflammation. These mixes help to improve insulin sensitivity, control blood sugar levels, and minimize the risk of developing type 2 diabetes.

We have thoughtfully included a variety of tea recipes in this book. That is both delicious and profitable for people with diabetes. Wide tea varieties, including black, green, white, natural, and organic product teas, are used in our recipes. Also, we have included recipes that include a variety of ingredients, such as cinnamon, ginger, turmeric, and other ingredients whose beneficial effects on blood sugar levels have all been demonstrated. We will take care of you whether you're looking for a soothing cup of tea to help you relax after a routine day or a rejuvenating cold tea for a warm summer evening. Our recipes are simple to follow and use ingredients that are easily found at your local grocery or online.

As a result, whether you're a tea connoisseur or new to the world of tea, This book is a great resource for anybody wishing to include tea in their diabetes treatment strategy. You may sip tea and work toward greater health and well-being with the help of our assortment of delectable and nutritious tea recipes.

Chapter 1

Understanding Diabetes and the Role of Tea

What is Diabetes?

Millions of individuals throughout the world suffer from diabetes, which is a common medical ailment. The World Diabetes Federation estimates that 537 million people worldwide will have diabetes by the year 2021. Although it can happen at any age, the illness is most prevalent in those over the age of 45.

Type 1 diabetes, Type 2 diabetes, gestational diabetes, and prediabetes are just a few of the several kinds of diabetes. With type 1 diabetes, the body lacks insulin because the immune system erroneously targets and kills the cells in the pancreas that make it. When the body develops insulin resistance and the pancreas is unable to generate enough insulin to overcome this resistance, Type 2 Diabetes, which is more prevalent, results. Pregnancy-related diabetes is known as gestational diabetes, whereas pre-diabetes is a disease in which blood sugar levels are elevated but not high enough to be categorized as diabetes.

Obesity, a sedentary lifestyle, family history, high blood pressure, high cholesterol, and gestational diabetes are all risk factors for the disease. Routine checkups and screenings are crucial in order To find out the problem early and treat it well, routine checkups and screenings are crucial.

Diabetes must be managed using a multifaceted strategy that includes medication, lifestyle changes, and dietary adjustments. Blood sugar levels can be controlled by eating a balanced diet rich in fruits, vegetables, lean protein, and whole grains. As tea includes substances that have been demonstrated to increase insulin sensitivity, reduce blood sugar levels, and have other positive effects, including tea in a diabetes control strategy, can also be useful. Lessen the likelihood of developing type 2 diabetes by lowering blood sugar levels. Ultimately, diabetes is a significant medical illness that has to be managed and monitored carefully. People with diabetes may live healthy, meaningful lives with the correct approach and support.

How Does Tea Affect Blood Sugar Levels?

- Theaflavins, catechins, and caffeine are just a few of the substances found in tea that might have an impact on blood sugar levels. Though not completely understood, the precise process by which tea influences blood sugar levels is yet unknown.

- Caffeine is a stimulant that can improve insulin sensitivity, allowing the body to utilize insulin to carry glucose into the cells more efficiently. This may aid in lowering blood sugar levels and enhancing glucose management.
- Tea contains antioxidants called catechins, which are most prevalent in green tea.

According to research, catechins may help raise insulin sensitivity, boost muscle glucose absorption, and decrease liver glucose synthesis, all of which may help lower blood sugar levels.

- Black tea has a specific kind of antioxidant called theaflavins. By preventing the action of enzymes involved in the synthesis of glucose, they have been proven to increase insulin sensitivity and lower blood glucose levels.

Moreover, tea consumption can help lower blood sugar levels. Tea consumption can help reduce cravings for sugary beverages and is a low-calorie approach to remaining hydrated. This can support more consistent blood sugar levels throughout the day and help reduce blood sugar spikes.

Overall, there is evidence to suggest that using tea in a diabetes care plan may enhance glucose control, even though the additional study is required to completely understand the effects of tea on blood sugar levels. It is crucial to remember that tea should be used as part of a complete diabetes care plan and not as a replacement for medicine or other diabetes control techniques.

Benefits of Tea for Diabetes

People with diabetes may benefit from tea in a number of ways, including:

1. **Increased insulin sensitivity,** increased muscle glucose absorption, and decreased liver glucose synthesis are all effects of the chemicals found in tea that have been demonstrated to improve insulin sensitivity, lower blood sugar levels, and enhance glucose management.

2. **Decreased risk of type 2 diabetes development:** Much research has revealed a link between frequent tea drinking and a lower risk of type 2 diabetes development. For instance, research indicated that consuming at least three cups of tea daily was linked to a 16% lower risk of type 2 diabetes. This study was published in the Archives of Internal Medicine.

3. **Better cardiovascular health:** Diabetes puts patients at risk for cardiovascular disease because it raises blood pressure and cholesterol levels in many diabetics. Tea includes

substances that have been demonstrated to lower blood pressure and improve cholesterol levels, such as catechins, which may assist in enhancing cardiovascular health.

4. **Anti-inflammatory** properties: Diabetes is linked to chronic inflammation, which can worsen kidney disease, heart disease, and nerve damage, among other consequences. Epigallocatechin gallate (EGCG), a chemical found in tea with anti-inflammatory characteristics, may assist in lessening

inflammation and safeguarding against problems.

5. **Tea may offer advantages for weight control** because obesity is a significant risk factor for type 2 diabetes. For instance, research indicated that intake of green tea was linked to decreased body weight, body mass index (BMI), and waist circumference in those who were overweight or obese.

6. **Enhanced cognitive function:** Diabetes is linked to a higher risk of dementia and cognitive

decline. Compounds in tea may help prevent age-related cognitive decline and enhance cognitive performance. For instance, a study indicated that older persons who regularly drank tea had a higher cognitive function, according to research published in the Journal of Nutrition, Health, and Aging.

7. **Antioxidant qualities:** Diabetes is linked to increased oxidative stress, which can lead to consequences including cardiovascular disease, renal disease, and nerve damage. Antioxidants in tea, such as polyphenols, may help defend against oxidative stress and

lower the likelihood of problems.

8. **Decreased risk of diabetic retinopathy**: One of the complications of diabetes, diabetic retinopathy can cause visual loss. Tea includes substances that have been found to enhance blood flow to the retina and protect against oxidative stress, such as epicatechin in green tea, which may help prevent diabetic retinopathy.

9. Gut health is improved: Diabetes is linked to a higher risk of gastrointestinal issues such as gastro paresis and irritable bowel syndrome. Tea includes substances that have been demonstrated to have prebiotic effects and stimulate the growth of good gut bacteria, such as catechins, which have been shown to aid gut health.

10. **Reduced risk of other illnesses:** Diabetes is linked to a higher risk of illnesses, including cancer, Alzheimer's disease, and Parkinson's disease. Tea includes substances that have been found

to have anti-cancer and neuroprotective characteristics, such as catechins and theaflavins, which may help lower the chance of developing these disorders.

Generally, tea has a wide range of positive effects on diabetes. Yet, it's crucial to remember that not all teas offer the same health benefits, and some varieties can have extra sugars or other additives that could harm blood sugar regulation. When introducing tea into a diabetic control plan, it is crucial to identify teas that have little to no added sugar and to consult a healthcare professional.

Chapter 2

Brewing the Perfect Cup of Tea

Tea Types and Varieties

There are several kinds and variations of tea, each having a special flavor, scent, and health advantages. The following are some of the popular varieties of tea:

- **Black tea:** Black tea is produced by fermenting and oxidizing Camellia sinensis plant leaves. It tastes strong and powerful and is frequently consumed with milk and sugar. Black tea includes antioxidants and caffeine, which may be good for blood sugar regulation, brain function, and heart health.

- **Green tea:** green tea is produced from the steamed or pan-fried leaves of the Camellia sinensis plant. It frequently tastes green and vegetal and is consumed straight or with a splash of lemon. Green tea may help with weight loss, cardiovascular health, and cognitive function since it includes caffeine and a lot of antioxidants.

- **White tea:** White tea is produced by drying and minimally processing young Camellia sinensis plant leaves and buds. It frequently tastes best when consumed simply or with a little honey and has a delicate, flowery flavor. White tea includes antioxidants and caffeine, which may be good for the skin, the heart, and the mind.

- **Oolong tea:** Oolong tea is produced by partly fermenting and oxidizing Camellia sinensis plant leaves. It often tastes better without milk or sugar and has a rich, deep flavor. Caffeine and antioxidants in oolong tea may help with weight loss, cardiovascular health, and bone health.

- **Herbal tea:** Rather than the Camellia sinensis plant, a variety of herbs, fruits, and flowers are used to make herbal tea. It is available in a broad range of tastes and may be consumed either hot or cold. Depending on the particular herbs used, herbal teas are frequently caffeine-free and may offer a range of health advantages.

Herbal teas that are well-liked include:

- **Chamomile:** chamomile tea has a delicate, flowery taste. It is frequently savored as a tea before night and may be beneficial for unwinding and sleeping.
- **Peppermint:** peppermint tea has a cooling, minty flavor. It could be advantageous for respiratory and digestive health.
- **Rooibos:** Rooibos tea has a sweet, nutty flavor. It is frequently consumed as a caffeine-free substitute for black

or green tea and may be good for bone and blood sugar regulation.

- Black tea that has been flavored with bergamot orange oil is known as Earl Grey tea. It tastes strongly of flowers and is frequently consumed with milk and sugar. The caffeine and antioxidants in earl grey tea may help with heart health and brain function.

- Green tea that has been flavored with jasmine blossoms is known as jasmine tea. It frequently tastes best when consumed simply or with a little honey and has a delicate, flowery flavor. Caffeine and antioxidants in jasmine tea may help with relaxation and stress reduction.

- **Masala Chai:** Black tea, milk, and a mixture of spices, including cinnamon, cardamom, and ginger, are commonly used to make masala chai, a spicy drink. It has a smoky, warming flavor that is frequently paired with a drizzle of honey. Masala chai includes antioxidants and caffeine, which may help with blood sugar regulation and digestive health.

- **Fruit and Herbal Blends:** Those who want caffeine-free teas choose fruit and herbal mixes. These mixtures can have a variety of tastes and possible health advantages. They can be produced using a number of fruits, herbs, and spices. Raspberry tea, lemon ginger tea, and hibiscus tea are some examples of well-liked fruit and herbal mixes.

While picking a tea for diabetes, it is crucial to pay attention to any added sugars or sweets. Several flavored teas and blends have added sugars or artificial sweeteners, which can significantly affect blood sugar regulation. Look for teas that are marked as "unsweetened" or "no added sugar" to avoid these additional sugars, and if desired, try a little amount of honey or a natural sugar replacement like stevia.\

Ultimately, there is a tea to fit every taste preference and health need, thanks to the large range of tea varieties and mixes that are available. Those with diabetes can take advantage of tea's numerous potential health advantages while simultaneously maintaining good blood sugar management by trying out various sorts and flavors.

How to Brew Tea

Tea brewing is an easy task that can be mastered with practice. These are some general recommendations for making tea:

❖ **Heat the Water:** Heating the water to the proper temperature is the first step in making tea. It's crucial to consider the sort of tea you're brewing since different kinds of tea require different water temperatures. For instance, black tea is normally made using water that has been heated to boiling (212°F), whereas green tea is typically made with water that has been cooked to about 175–180°F. A good general rule of thumb is to boil the water, let it cool for a few minutes, and then pour it over the tea.

❖ Measure out the necessary amount of tea after the water has been heated to the proper temperature. Use around one teaspoon of loose-leaf tea or one tea bag per 8 ounces of water as a general guideline.

❖ Put the tea in the teapot, a tea bag, a tea infuser, or both too steep. The tea should steep for the indicated period of time after being covered with warm water. As a general guideline, green tea should be steeped for 2-3 minutes, black tea for 3-5 minutes, and herbal tea for 5-7 minutes. Steeping lengths vary based on the kind of tea.

❖ Remove the tea infuser or tea bags from the tea and filter the liquid to get rid of any loose tea leaves or other particles before serving. If preferred, you can serve the tea hot or cold.

The brewing procedure may vary slightly based on the type of tea and individual tastes, which is crucial to mention. For instance, some people could choose to steep their tea for a shorter or longer amount of time, or they might prefer a stronger or weaker brew. You may discover the brewing technique that suits your needs and tastes with a little experimentation and practice.

Tips for Enhancing Flavor

There are various suggestions you may attempt if you want to improve the flavor of your tea:

❖ **Squeeze in a little lemon juice:** Squeezing a little lemon juice into your tea can help to brighten the flavor and provide a little acidity. In addition to vitamin C and other healthy nutrients, lemon also has these properties.

❖ **Add a little honey or natural sweetener** if you want your tea a little sweeter: If you like your tea a little sweeter, think about adding a little honey or natural sweetener, such as stevia or agave. Be careful how much sweetener you use since too much might make it difficult to manage blood sugar levels.

❖ **Try out various herbs and spices:** Adding herbs and spices to your tea may give the flavor more depth and complexity. Ginger, cinnamon, cardamom, and mint are a few well-liked herbs and spices to explore.

❖ **Utilize top-notch tea:** Using top-notch tea may help your beverage taste and smell better. Choose teas that are manufactured with complete tea leaves and are devoid of additives and artificial flavors.

❖ **Use the right length of time to brew the tea;** either too much or too little time might have a negative effect on the flavor. Ensure that you steep your tea according to the required time.

❖ **Employ water that is the proper temperature;** using water that is either too hot or too cold might affect how your tea tastes. Use water that has been heated to the right temperature for the sort of tea you are drinking.

You may discover fresh and inventive methods to improve the flavor of your tea and make your tea-drinking experience more pleasurable by experimenting with these tricks and suggestions.

Chapter 3

Black Tea Recipes

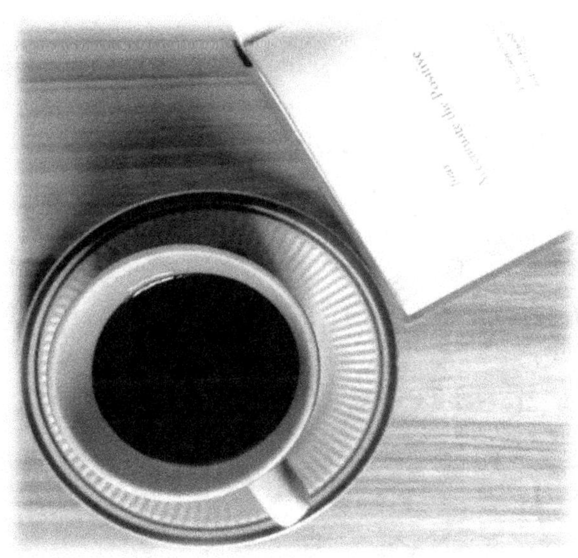

Classic Black Tea;

One of the most well-liked and regularly eaten tea varieties worldwide is traditional black tea. It is produced from the Camellia sinensis plant's leaves and is often subjected to greater levels of oxidation than other varieties of tea, giving it its distinctively black color and powerful flavor.

Black tea may be prepared hot or cold and is delicious either alone or with a little milk or sweetness. It is frequently used as the foundation for flavored teas and tea mixes.

In addition to its robust flavor and adaptability, black tea is said to provide a number of health advantages. Black tea, for instance, has antioxidants called polyphenols that have been demonstrated to enhance heart health, decrease cholesterol levels, as well as encourage normal blood sugar levels.

Caffeine, another ingredient in black tea, can aid in increasing energy and mental clarity. Caffeine use must be monitored, though, since too much of it can have unfavorable consequences, including jitters, anxiety, and disturbed sleep.

In general, traditional black tea is a well-liked beverage that provides a rich and pleasing flavor in addition to certain health advantages. Black tea is a common item in the collections of many tea lovers, whether it is consumed alone or as a component of a tea mix.

Here is a straightforward home recipe for classic black tea:

Ingredients:

- One teaspoon of black tea bags or black tea leaves
- Water, 8 to 10 ounces
- Milk, honey, or other sweeteners are optional.

Instructions:

1. In a saucepan or kettle, bring water to a boil.
2. Black loose-leaf tea should be added to a teapot or tea infuser. Just put the tea bag in the mug if you are using one.

3. After adding the boiling water to the tea, let it steep for three to five minutes.
4. Take off the tea bag or infuser from the mug or teapot.
5. If desired, add milk and/or sugar to taste.
6. Take pleasure in your freshly prepared Cup of black tea.

Note: The steeping time can vary depending on personal preference and the type of black tea you are using. Experiment with different steeping times to find your perfect Cup of tea.

Earl Grey Tea

It is unknown who named Earl Grey tea; however, Charles Grey, the 2nd Earl Grey, and a former British prime minister are said to have received the tea as a gift. The flavor of Earl Grey tea is unique and aromatic and has flowery and lemony undertone. It may be brewed hot or cold and is frequently served straight, with a little milk or sugar, or both.

Earl Grey tea is renowned for its distinct flavor as well as a number of purported health advantages. For instance, the black tea used to make Earl Grey includes anti-inflammatory antioxidants that can benefit general health. Since bergamot oil is thought to contain antibacterial, antifungal, and anti-inflammatory qualities, it may also have health advantages when used to flavor Earl Grey.

Just steep a tea bag or loose-leaf tea in boiling water for 3-5 minutes, or until the required strength is attained, to prepare Earl Grey tea. If desired, add milk and/or sugar to taste. Earl Grey tea is a tasty and invigorating beverage that has been savored by tea connoisseurs all over the world for generations, whether as a morning pick-me-up or an afternoon pleasure.

For Earl Grey tea, here are two recipes:

Typical Ingredients for Earl Grey Tea

- One teaspoon Earl Grey tea bags or one teaspoon Earl Grey loose-leaf tea
- Water, 8 to 10 ounces
- Milk, honey, or other sweeteners are optional.

Instructions:

1. In a saucepan or kettle, bring water to a boil.
2. Use a teapot or tea infuser to add loose-leaf Earl Grey tea. Just put the tea bag in the mug if you are using one.

3. After adding the boiling water to the tea, let it steep for three to five minutes.

4. Take off the tea bag or infuser from the mug or teapot.
5. If desired, add milk and/or sugar to taste.

Recipe for Earl Grey Latte:

Ingredients:

- One bag of Earl Grey tea
- Milk, 6 to 8 ounces (dairy or non-dairy)
- Sweetener to taste is optional.

Instructions:

1. In a small saucepan over medium heat, warm the milk until it starts to steam. Never boil.
2. The boiling milk should now include an Earl Grey tea bag. Let it steep for three to five minutes.
3. Pour the milk into a blender after removing the tea bag.
4. The milk should be blended on high for 20 to 30 seconds or until it foams.
5. In a cup, pour the frothed milk.
6. If desired, add sweetener to taste.
7. Make a different cup of Earl Grey tea according to the traditional directions above.

8. In the mug with the foamy milk, pour the brewed tea.

9. Tea and milk should be combined with a spoon.

Take pleasure in your tasty Earl Grey latte!

Note: If you don't have a blender, you may make foam with a frother or by hand-whisking warm milk.

Chai Tea

The popular spiced tea known as chai, commonly referred to as masala chai has its roots in India. Black tea is frequently steeped in a blend of milk, water, and other spices, including cinnamon, ginger, cardamom, and cloves, to make chai tea. The end product is a creamy, fragrant, spicy beverage that is frequently served with honey or sugar added for sweetness.

In India, where it has been enjoyed for many years as a ceremonial and medicinal beverage, chai tea has a long and illustrious history. The precise recipe for chai tea might vary based on the locale and the maker's personal preferences, but the essential components are often black tea, milk, water, and a mix of spices. Chai tea has a great taste and may also have a number of health advantages. Black tea, for instance, has antioxidants that may boost general health and lessen inflammation. The spices used in chai tea are also said to provide a variety of health advantages, including enhancing heart health, lowering inflammation, and assisting with digestion.

You will need a few simple materials, some time, and patience to prepare chai tea. To help you get started here is a traditional chai tea recipe:

Ingredients:

- 2-cups of water
- Two sticks of cinnamon

- 6-8 pods of cardamom, gently crushed
- 6 to 8 cloves whole
- 1-2 inches of freshly peeled and sliced ginger
- 2-4 bags of black tea
- Milk, two cups (dairy or non-dairy)
- To taste, use sugar or honey.

Instructions:

1. Bring the water to a boil in a small saucepan.
2. To the saucepan, add the cloves, cinnamon sticks, cardamom pods, and ginger slices.

3. Stirring occasionally, lower the heat to a simmer, and cook the spices for ten to fifteen minutes.

4. Steep the black tea bags in the kettle for 3 to 5 minutes after adding them.

5. Simmer the mixture after adding the milk to the saucepan.

6. To enable the flavors to merge, turn off the heat and let the pot sit for 5–10 minutes.

7. To get the spices and tea bags out of the chai tea mixture, strain it over a fine-mesh sieve.

8. If desired, add honey or sugar to taste.

The chai tea should be served hot.

Masala Chai Tea

Masala chai tea, commonly referred to as spiced chai tea, is a delectable and fragrant brew that has its roots in India. Black tea is used to make this tasty tea, which is often served with honey or sugar and a variety of fragrant spices, including cardamom, cinnamon, ginger, and cloves.

This is a simple homemade recipe for traditional masala chai tea:

Ingredients:

- 2-cups of water
- 2-4 black tea bags or black tea leaves

- a cup of milk (dairy or non-dairy)
- 1-stick of cinnamon
- 4 to 5 entire, lightly crushed green cardamom pods
- Sliced and peeled fresh ginger, 1 inch long.
- 2 to 3 entire cloves
- 1 to 2 tablespoons of black pepper, loose
- Fennel seeds, loose leaf, 1 to 2 tablespoons

Instructions:

1. Bring the water to a boil in a medium-sized saucepan.

2. The water should be simmered with the cinnamon stick, cardamom pods, ginger, cloves, black pepper, and fennel seeds for around five minutes.
3. Black tea bags or loose leaves should be added to the kettle and steeped for three to five minutes.
4. After adding the milk, boil the mixture for an additional two to three minutes.
5. After taking the pot off the heat, drain the tea mixture to get rid of the spices and tea leaves.
6. If desired, taste and add more sugar or honey.

Enjoy the masala chai tea after serving it hot!

Chapter 4

Green Tea Recipes

Classic Green Tea

The globe over, people enjoy the famous and nutritious beverage known as green tea. This tea is prepared from the Camellia sinensis plant's leaves and is a great source of antioxidants and other health-improving substances.

This is a traditional green tea recipe that is simple to prepare at home:

Ingredients:

- one water cup
- 1-2 tablespoons of loose-leaf green tea or one green tea bag
- Slice of lemon, optional

Instructions:

1. Bring the water to a boil in a small saucepan.
2. When the water has boiled, turn off the heat and let it cool for a few seconds.

3. The green tea bag or loose green tea should be added to the kettle and steeped for two to three minutes.
4. Take out the tea bag or use a fine-mesh sieve to separate the tea leaves from the tea.
5. Add honey and a squeeze of lemon juice to taste, if preferred.
6. Enjoy the hot green tea after serving!

Reminder: Avoid overstepping green tea, as it might become bitter. Also, the water should be about 175°F (80°C) in temperature since boiling water might burn the delicate green tea leaves. Your individual taste preferences may be accommodated by adjusting the brewing time and temperature.

Matcha Tea

Due to its distinctive flavor and many health advantages, matcha tea, a form of green tea, has been more popular in recent years. Shade-grown green tea leaves are used to manufacture this tea, which is created from a vivid green powder that is whisked into hot water to create a frothy and tasty beverage.

An easy recipe for preparing matcha tea at home is provided below:

Ingredients:

- A smidge of matcha powder
- Hot water, 2 ounces (not boiling)
- Milk, 6 ounces (dairy or non-dairy)
- Sweetener, if desired (optional)

Instructions:

1. To get rid of any clumps, sift the matcha powder into a small dish.
2. After the matcha is completely dissolved and foamy, add the hot water to the bowl and whisk the mixture briskly with a bamboo whisk or a frother.

3. The milk should be heated in a microwave or a small saucepan to the appropriate temperature.
4. Pour the heated milk over the foamy matcha mixture into the Cup.
5. The sweetener can be added and stirred if desired.

Enjoy the hot matcha tea after serving!

Please take note that using water that is too hot can burn the delicate matcha powder and produce a harsh flavor.

Sencha Tea

Sencha tea is a popular variety of Japanese green tea because of its flavorful appeal and a host of health advantages. It is created from Camellia sinensis plant leaves that are cultivated in direct sunlight and then steamed to avoid oxidation, giving it a vivid green color and a flavor that is both fresh and grassy.

This is a traditional sencha tea recipe:

Ingredients:

- 8 ounces of water and one teaspoon of sencha tea leaves
- Slice of lemon, optional
- Oh, and optional

Instructions:

1. Using a small saucepan or kettle, bring water to a boil.
2. Let the water cool to a temperature of around 175°F (80°C) over the course of 2–3 minutes.
3. Put the sencha tea leaves into an infuser or teapot.
4. Tea leaves should be covered with boiling water, and they should steep for 1 to 2 minutes.
5. Take off the tea leaves from the infuser or teapot.
6. Add honey and a squeeze of lemon juice to taste, if preferred.

Enjoy the sencha tea after pouring it into a cup.

Note: If you want a stronger flavor, brew sencha tea for longer than two minutes. It's crucial to avoid using boiling water since it might harm the delicate tea leaves and produce a harsh flavor. Sencha

Genmaicha Tea

Japanese green tea called genmaicha is flavored with toasted brown rice. It is frequently used as a soothing and warming beverage and has a distinctive flavor and scent that is both nutty and earthy.

Here is a straightforward recipe for genmaicha tea:

Ingredients:

- Tea leaves from genmaicha, 1 tbsp
- Water, 8 ounces
- optional roasted brown rice

Instructions:

1. Using a small saucepan or kettle, bring water to a boil.
2. Let the water cool to a temperature of around 175°F (80°C) over the course of 2–3 minutes.
3. Use an infuser or teapot to add the genmaicha tea leaves.

4. The tea should steep for two to three minutes after being added to the boiling water.

5. Take off the tea leaves from the infuser or teapot.

6. For a more nutty flavor and scent, you can, if you want, add a few bits of brown rice that has been roasted to the tea.

Genmaicha tea should be poured into a cup and enjoyed!

Note: You can modify the quantity of water and tea leaves to suit your own taste preferences. Genmaicha tea may be consumed cold as well by steeping the tea leaves in ice.

Chapter 5

White Tea Recipes

Silver Needle Tea

Chinese white tea, known as "Silver Needle," is renowned for its delicate flavor and a host of health advantages. The young, unopened buds of the Camellia sinensis plant, which give the tea its unique look, are used to make this beverage.

The following is a recipe for silver needle tea:

Ingredients:

- One tablespoon of tea leaves with silver needles
- Water, 8 ounces
- optional honey or lemon wedge

Instructions:

1. Using a small saucepan or kettle, bring water to a boil.
2. Let the water cool to a temperature of around 175°F (80°C) over the course of 2–3 minutes.

3. Teapot or infuser should be filled with silver needle tea leaves.

4. The tea should steep for two to three minutes after being added to the boiling water.

5. Take off the tea leaves from the infuser or teapot.

6. If preferred, season with a squeeze of lemon juice or a drizzle of honey.

Enjoy the silver needle tea after pouring it into a cup.

Since boiling water might harm the delicate tea leaves and produce a harsh flavor, Silver Needle tea should be steeped at a lower temperature than other teas. If you want a stronger flavor, brew the tea for longer than 2-3 minutes. By steeping the tea leaves in cold water for an extended amount of time and including ice cubes just before serving, silver needle tea may also be savored cold.

White Peony Tea

Bai Mu Dan, another name for white peony tea, is a kind of Chinese white tea renowned for its delicate and mild flavor. It is created from the Camellia sinensis plant's unopened buds and the first two leaves, which are allowed to naturally wither and dry in the sun or in a warm indoor atmosphere.

The following is a recipe for white peony tea:

Ingredients:

- one-fourth cup of white peony tea leaves
- Water, 8 ounces

optional honey or agave syrup

Instructions:

1. Using a small saucepan or kettle, bring water to a boil.
2. Let the water cool to a temperature of around 175°F

(80°C) over the course of 2–3 minutes.

3. Teapot or infuser with white peony tea leaves added.
4. The tea should steep for two to three minutes after being added to the boiling water.
5. Take off the tea leaves from the infuser or teapot.
6. Add honey or agave syrup to taste, if preferred.
7. Enjoy the white peony tea after pouring it into a cup.

As opposed to other teas, white peony tea should be steeped at a lower temperature since boiling water might scald delicate tea leaves and provide a harsh flavor. If you want a stronger flavor, brew the tea for longer than 2-3 minutes. By letting the tea leaves soak in cold water for a longer amount of time, white peony tea may also be drunk cold.

Jasmine Silver Needle Tea

Chinese white tea, known as "Jasmine Silver Needle," has a distinct and aromatic flavor since it is flavored with jasmine blossoms. Young, unopened Camellia sinensis plant buds coated in delicate white hairs are used to make it. Fresh jasmine flowers are then added to give them flavor and scent.

The following is the recipe for Jasmine Silver Needle tea:

Ingredients:

- One tablespoon silver needle jasmine tea leaves
- Water, 8 ounces
- sugar or honey, optional

Instructions:

1. Using a small saucepan or kettle, bring water to a boil.

2. Let the water cool to a temperature of around 175°F (80°C) over the course of 2–3 minutes.

3. To a teapot or infuser, add the jasmine silver needle tea leaves.

4. The tea should steep for two to three minutes after being added to the boiling water.

5. Take off the tea leaves from the infuser or teapot.

6. Add a drizzle of honey or sugar to taste, if preferred.

Enjoy the jasmine silver needle tea after pouring it into a cup.

Since boiling water might harm the delicate tea leaves and produce a harsh flavor, Jasmine Silver Needle tea should be steeped at a lower temperature than other teas. If you want a stronger flavor, brew the tea for longer than 2-3 minutes. By steeping the tea leaves in cold water for an extended amount of time and including ice cubes just before serving, Jasmine Silver Needle tea may also be savored cold.

Chapter 6

Herbal Tea Recipes

Chamomile Tea

Tea produced from dried chamomile flowers is known as chamomile tea. It has a pleasant, tranquil flavor that is frequently appreciated for its calming properties. In addition to its numerous health advantages, chamomile tea is also renowned for relaxing the body and mind.

The following is a recipe for chamomile tea:

Ingredients:

- One teaspoon of chamomile flowers, dried
- Water, 8 ounces
- Lemon or honey, optional

Instructions:

1. Using a small pot or kettle, bring water to a boil.
2. Dried chamomile flowers should be placed in a teapot or infuser.
3. The chamomile flowers should steep in the heated water for around five minutes.

4. Remove the chamomile flowers from the infuser or teapot.

5. Add honey or a squeeze of lemon to taste, if preferred.

Enjoy the chamomile tea after pouring it into a cup.

Note: You can drink chamomile tea, either hot or cold. You can steep the chamomile flowers for a longer time if you desire a stronger flavor. After a long day, chamomile tea is a wonderful way to relax. It can also be used as a home cure for insomnia and moderate anxiety.

Ginger Tea

Ginger root or ginger powder is used to make ginger tea, a herbal beverage. It has a warm, spicy flavor and is well-liked for its various health advantages, which include promoting healthy digestion and lowering inflammation.

The following is a recipe for ginger tea:

Ingredients:

- Two glasses of water
- Two teaspoons of ginger powder or 2 inches of freshly peeled and sliced ginger
- Lemon or honey, optional

Instructions:

1. In a small pot or kettle, bring 2 cups of water to a rolling boil.
2. Simmer the mixture while adding the ginger powder or fresh ginger root slices.
3. Let the ginger simmer for ten to fifteen minutes.
4. After taking the pot from the heat, give it some time to cool.
5. In a mug, strain the tea.
6. Add honey or a squeeze of lemon to taste, if preferred.

Cheers to your ginger tea!

Note: Depending on how spicy you like your tea, you can change how much ginger is used in this recipe.

You can increase the ginger in your tea if you prefer it quite spicy. On chilly days or to calm an upset stomach, ginger tea is a terrific way to stay warm. As a natural treatment for cold and flu symptoms, it is also an option.

Turmeric Tea

The dried turmeric plant roots are used to make turmeric tea, a herbal beverage. It tastes warm and earthy and has a long list of health advantages, including lowering inflammation and enhancing the immune system.

The following is a recipe for turmeric tea:

Ingredients:

- Two glasses of water
- 1/2 teaspoon of turmeric powder or one teaspoon of freshly grated turmeric root
- 1/2 teaspoon of ginger powder or one teaspoon of freshly grated ginger root
- One teaspoon of maple syrup or honey (optional)
- One teaspoon of lemon juice, fresh (optional)

Instructions:

1. In a small pot or kettle, bring 2 cups of water to a rolling boil.
2. Stir in the freshly grated ginger and turmeric roots, then lower the heat to a simmer.
3. Let the ginger and turmeric simmer for 10 to 15 minutes.
4. After taking the pot from the heat, give it some time to cool.
5. In a mug, strain the tea.
6. To taste, add a squeeze of fresh lemon juice and a drizzle of honey or maple syrup.

Enjoy your turmeric tea after a thorough stirring!

Be careful when handling fresh turmeric root or turmeric powder since it can stain clothing and surfaces. The health advantages of turmeric can easily be incorporated into your diet by drinking turmeric tea.

Rooibos Tea

The leaves of the Rooibos plant, which is indigenous to South Africa, are used to make Rooibos tea, commonly referred to as red bush tea. It is a well-liked substitute for conventional tea and coffee since it has a sweet, nutty flavor and contains no caffeine.

The following is a recipe for Rooibos tea:

Ingredients:

- Two glasses of water
- 1-2 teaspoons of loose Rooibos tea or 2-3 Rooibos tea bags, as desired. Honey or lemon (optional)

Instructions:

1. In a small pot or kettle, bring 2 cups of water to a rolling boil.
2. Then turn down the heat to a simmer and add the Rooibos tea bags or loose tea to the saucepan.
3. Simmer the tea for 5 to 7 minutes.

4. After taking the pot from the heat, give it some time to cool.

5. In a mug, strain the tea.

6. If preferred, season with a squeeze of lemon juice or a drizzle of honey.

7. Mix thoroughly, then savor your Rooibos tea.

Very sweet by nature, Rooibos tea doesn't require much sweetening. It can be consumed hot or cold, and you can use it as a base for herbal concoctions by incorporating cinnamon, ginger, or mint.

Many health advantages of Rooibos tea include lowering inflammation and enhancing heart health. Also, it has a lot of

antioxidants, which can lessen the
risk of free radicals harming cells.

Chapter 7

Fruit Tea Recipes

Hibiscus Tea

The dried blossoms of the tropical-native Hibiscus sabdariffa plant are used to make the popular herbal beverage known as hibiscus tea. It tastes tangy and cranberry-like and is good warmed or cold.

The following is a recipe for hibiscus tea:

Ingredients:

- Two glasses of water

- Dried hibiscus blossoms, half a cup
- To taste, honey or agave syrup (optional)
- Slices of lime or lemon for decoration (optional)

Instructions:

1. In a medium pot, bring 2 cups of water to a boil.
2. Then turn down the heat to a simmer and add the dried hibiscus blossoms to the pot.
3. Let the tea simmer for 5-7 minutes while stirring now and then.

4. After taking the pot from the heat, give it some time to cool.
5. Then put the tea in a big jug or pitcher, and strain it.
6. Add honey or agave syrup to taste, if preferred.
7. Tea should be chilled in the fridge for at least 30 minutes.
8. If desired, top the hibiscus tea with ice and garnish with lemon or lime slices.

The numerous health advantages of hibiscus tea include its capacity to enhance cholesterol levels, lower blood pressure, and reduce inflammation. Moreover, it has a lot of vitamin C and antioxidants, which can strengthen the immune system and stop free radicals from causing cell damage. Moreover, hibiscus tea has been demonstrated to possess diuretic effects, which can aid in the body's removal of extra water and impurities.

Peach Tea

Peach tea is a tasty and reviving drink that combines the tea's mild bitterness with the sweetness of ripe peaches. It is a terrific way to quench your thirst on a hot summer day and maybe drunk hot or cold.

The following is a recipe for peach tea:

Ingredients:

- 4 cups of liquid
- Four bags of black tea
- Two pitted and sliced ripe peaches
- 1/4 cup of sugar or honey
- Fresh peach slices as a garnish (optional)

Instructions:

1. In a medium pot, bring 4 cups of water to a boil.

2. Steep the black tea bags into the pot for 5-7 minutes after adding them.

3. Take out the tea bags, then wait a few minutes for the tea to cool.

4. Simmer the sliced peaches in the stew for ten to fifteen minutes.

5. After straining the tea into a sizable pitcher or jug, turn off the heat.

6. Add the sugar or honey and stir until combined.

7. Tea should be chilled in the fridge for at least 30 minutes.

8. If preferred, top the peach tea with ice and garnish with fresh peach slices.

Vitamin C, which can aid in strengthening the immune system and stave off cell damage brought on by free radicals, is abundant in peach tea. Moreover, it has a lot of antioxidants, which can help prevent cancer and heart disease, as well as other chronic illnesses. Peach tea has also been demonstrated to have anti-inflammatory qualities, which can aid in reducing pain and inflammation.

Apple Cinnamon Tea

A warm and soothing beverage, apple cinnamon tea is ideal for chilly fall days or comfortable nights at home. Black tea is infused with the aromas of crisp apples and comforting cinnamon spice to create this beverage. The following is a recipe for homemade apple cinnamon tea:

Ingredients:

- 4 cups of liquid
- Four bags of black tea
- Few cinnamon sticks
- Sliced thinly, one huge apple
- One tablespoon of maple syrup or honey (optional)

Instructions:

1. Bring 4 cups of water to a boil in a medium pot.

2. To the saucepan, add the black tea bags and cinnamon sticks. Steep for three to five minutes.

3. Add the sliced apple to the pot after removing the tea bags and cinnamon sticks.

4. Stir the tea for 10 to 15 minutes.

5. After straining the tea into a sizable pitcher or jug, turn off the heat.

6. If used, add honey or maple syrup to taste.

7. With a cinnamon stick and apple slice for decoration, serve the apple cinnamon tea hot.

Due to the fresh apples used in the recipe, apple cinnamon tea is a fantastic source of antioxidants and vitamin C. It has been demonstrated that cinnamon has anti-inflammatory qualities and that it can assist in controlling sugar levels. Black tea also contains caffeine, which may support increased energy and mental clarity. It's a terrific idea to warm up with this tasty and soothing tea on a chilly day or to enjoy it as a sweet treat in the evening.

Blueberry Tea

Both hot and cold drinks can be enjoyed with blueberry tea because it is so tasty and flavorful. A sweet and fruity beverage is produced by combining black tea with fresh or dried blueberries. The following is a recipe for homemade blueberry tea:

Ingredients:

- 4 cups of liquid
- Four bags of black tea
- 1 cup of blueberries, either fresh or frozen
- 1 to 2 tablespoons of maple syrup or honey (optional)

Instructions:

1. Bring 4 cups of water to a boil in a medium pot.

2. Blueberries and black tea bags should be added to the saucepan and steeped for 3-5 minutes.

3. Take off the tea bags, then strain the tea through a cheesecloth or sieve to get the blueberries out.

4. If desired, whisk in honey or maple syrup.

5. With fresh blueberries or lemon slices as a garnish, you may serve the blueberry tea hot, or you can let it cool and pour it over ice for a revitalizing iced tea.

The antioxidant content of blueberries is well recognized, and they are also a fantastic source of vitamins C and K. Caffeine, which is present in black tea, can aid in increasing stamina and mental clarity. The health advantages of blueberries can be enjoyed in a delightful and simple-to-make tea with blueberry tea.

Chapter 8

Iced Tea Recipes

Classic Iced Tea

For hot summer days, classic iced tea is a cooling and simple beverage to prepare. Here is a straightforward formula for creating authentic iced tea at home:

Ingredients:

- Six bags of black tea
- 8 cups of liquid
- 1 cup of sugar, granulated
- One sliced lemon (optional)

- brand-new mint leaves (optional)

Instructions:

1. Bring 8 cups of water to a boil in a big pot.
2. Six black tea bags should be added after taking the kettle off the heat.
3. Let the tea steep for 3 to 5 minutes, depending on the desired strength.
4. After removing the tea bags, mix in 1 cup of sugar until it has completely dissolved.
5. If preferred, include lemon slices and fresh mint leaves.

6. After the tea has cooled to room temperature, pour it into a pitcher and store it in the refrigerator until chilled.

7. Serve the classic iced tea over ice, garnished with more lemon slices and mint leaves, if preferred.

If you'd like, you can use a sugar substitute or change the amount of sugar to suit your tastes. Also, you can experiment with adding different flavors like peach or raspberry or switching to green tea from black tea. Any occasion is ideal for a pleasant, all-purpose beverage like classic iced tea.

Green Tea Mint Iced Tea

Cool and healthful beverage that is ideal for hot summer days is green tea and mint iced tea. An easy recipe for brewing green tea mint iced tea at home is provided below:

Ingredients:

- Four bags of green tea
- 8 cups of liquid
- A half-cup of honey
- Fresh mint leaves, 1/2 cup
- One sliced lemon (optional)

Instructions:

1. Bring 8 cups of water to a boil in a big pot.
2. Four green tea bags are added when the pot is taken off the heat.
3. Let the tea steep for 3 to 5 minutes, depending on the desired strength.
4. Tea bags should be taken out before adding honey and stirring until it dissolves.
5. Tea should be infused with fresh mint leaves and allowed to cool to room temperature.
6. Remove the mint leaves after the tea has cooled, then pour the tea into a pitcher.
7. For at least an hour, chill the tea.

8. If desired, top the green tea mint iced tea with lemon slices and serve over ice.

You can modify this recipe to your preferences. You can increase the honey if you like your tea sweeter. You can increase the number of mint leaves if you desire a stronger mint flavor. Iced tea with green tea and mint is a tasty and healthful year-round substitute for sweetened beverages.

Mango Iced Tea

A sweet and fruity drink ideal for summer is mango iced tea. An easy

recipe for homemade mango iced tea
is provided below:

Ingredients:

- Four bags of black tea
- 8 cups of liquid
- One mango that has been peeled
  and sliced.
- honey, 1/4 cup
- One sliced lemon (optional)

Instructions:

1. Bring 8 cups of water to a boil in
   a big pot.
2. Add four bags of black tea after
   turning off the heat in the kettle.

3. Let the tea steep for 3 to 5 minutes, depending on the desired strength.

4. Once the tea bags are out, add 1/4 cup of honey and stir until it has dissolved.

5. After the tea has cooled to room temperature, stir in the chopped mango.

6. Blend the tea and mango till smooth when it has cooled.

7. Blend the tea and mango till smooth when it has cooled.

8. Using a fine-mesh strainer, pour the blended tea into a pitcher.

9. For at least an hour, chill the tea.

10. If preferred, top the mango iced tea with lemon slices and serve over ice.

You can modify this recipe to your preferences. You can increase the honey if you like your tea sweeter. More mango or less tea can be added if you prefer a thicker consistency. A delightful and cool way to enjoy the summer sensations is with mango iced tea.

Lemon Ginger Iced Tea

The zesty flavors of lemon and ginger are combined with the coolness of iced tea to create the wonderful and energizing beverage known as lemon ginger iced tea. This is a home recipe for lemon ginger iced tea:

Ingredients:

- Four bags of black tea
- 8 cups of liquid
- A half-cup of honey
- Fresh lemon juice, 1/2 cup
- Sliced 1/4 cup fresh ginger
- An ice cube
- For garnish, use fresh mint leaves and lemon slices (optional)

Instructions:

1. Bring 8 cups of water to a boil in a big pot.
2. Add the ginger slices and four black tea bags after turning off the heat.

3. Let the tea steep for 3 to 5 minutes, depending on the desired strength.

4. After removing the tea bags and ginger, add 1/2 cup of honey and stir until it dissolves.

5. Stir in 1/2 cup of freshly squeezed lemon juice to the tea.

6. Tea should be allowed to reach room temperature before being chilled for at least an hour in the fridge.

7. Pour the iced tea over ice cubes and top with fresh mint leaves and lemon slices, if preferred, to serve.

Enjoy the cooling effects of this lemon ginger iced tea while reaping the advantages of ginger and lemon for your health. It can also be kept for up to five days in the refrigerator.

Conclusion

In conclusion, a diabetic's diet can benefit greatly from including tea. It is a wise choice for persons with diabetes due to its various health advantages, including boosting insulin sensitivity and lowering the chance of acquiring chronic illnesses. There is a tea type and flavor to suit every taste, thanks to the large variety of teas available. Diabetics can enjoy tasty and healthful tea options that can help them control their blood sugar levels and enhance their general health by utilizing the recipes and brewing methods in this book. So make a cup of your favorite tea and take advantage of all its health advantages!

A diabetic can also benefit from introducing tea into their daily routine by finding it to be calming and pleasurable. A brief period spent relaxing with a warm cup of tea can help lower stress levels and foster relaxation, both of which can benefit blood sugar levels. Many tea-related components, including ginger, turmeric, and hibiscus, have anti-inflammatory qualities that can help manage diabetes and other related health issues.

It's crucial to keep in mind that tea shouldn't be the only treatment for diabetes, and people should always talk to their doctor about their diet and treatment regimen. But, people with diabetes can take advantage of tea's many health-promoting qualities and enjoy a variety of delectable and refreshing flavors by including it in a balanced and healthy diet. All things considered, tea can be a useful complement to a diabetic's lifestyle and a delectable approach to promoting their health and well-being.

Glossary terms

Camellia sinensis: The plant species used to produce true teas, including black, green, white, oolong, and pu-erh tea.

Tisane: A tea-like beverage made from herbs, fruits, flowers, and other plant materials that are not from the Camellia Camellia sinensis: The plant species used to produce true teas, including black, green, white, oolong, and pu-erh tea.

Infusion: The process of steeping tea or other ingredients in hot water to extract their flavor and health benefits.

Steeping: The act of soaking tea leaves or other ingredients in hot water to extract their flavor and health benefits.

Oxidation: The natural process that occurs when tea leaves are exposed to air, which can change the flavor and color of the tea.

Fermentation: The process of allowing tea leaves to undergo controlled microbial fermentation, which can create unique flavors and aromas in certain types of tea, such as puerh tea.

Caffeine: A natural stimulant found in tea and coffee that can help increase alertness and concentration.

Theanine: An amino acid found in tea that can help promote relaxation and reduce stress and anxiety.

Antioxidants: Compounds found in tea that can help protect the body against oxidative stress and inflammation, which are associated with various chronic diseases.

Polyphenols: A group of antioxidants found in tea that can help regulate blood sugar levels, improve insulin sensitivity, and reduce the risk of developing type 2 diabetes.

Tannins: A group of bitter-tasting compounds found in tea that can bind with proteins and reduce the bioavailability of certain nutrients.

Brew time: The amount of time that tea leaves or other ingredients are steeped in hot water, which can impact the flavor, strength, and health benefits of the tea.

Water Temperature: The temperature of the hot water used to steep tea or other ingredients, which can impact the flavor, strength, and health benefits of the tea.

Teapot: A vessel used for brewing and serving tea, which can come in various sizes, shapes, and materials.

Teacup: A small Camellia sinensis: The plant species used to produce true teas, including black, green, white, oolong, and pu-erh tea.

Tisane: A tea-like beverage made from herbs, fruits, flowers, and other plant materials that are not from the Camellia sinensis plant.

Infusion: The process of steeping tea or other ingredients in hot water to extract their flavor and health benefits.

Steeping: The act of soaking tea leaves or other ingredients in hot water to extract their flavor and health benefits.

Oxidation: The natural process that occurs when tea leaves are exposed to air, which can change the flavor and color of the tea.

Fermentation: The process of allowing tea leaves to undergo controlled microbial fermentation, which can create unique flavors and aromas in certain types of tea, such as pu-erh tea.

Caffeine: A natural stimulant found in tea and coffee that can help increase alertness and concentration.

Theanine: An amino acid found in tea that can help promote relaxation and reduce stress and anxiety.

Antioxidants: Compounds found in tea that can help protect the body against oxidative stress and inflammation, which are associated with various chronic diseases.

Polyphenols: A group of antioxidants found in tea that can help regulate blood sugar levels, improve insulin sensitivity, and reduce the risk of developing type 2 diabetes.

Tannins: A group of bitter-tasting compounds found in tea that can bind with proteins and reduce the bioavailability of certain nutrients.

Brew time: The amount of time that tea leaves or other ingredients are steeped in hot water, which can impact the flavor, strength, and health benefits of the tea.

Water temperature: The temperature of the hot water used to steep tea or other ingredients, which can impact the flavor, strength, and health benefits of the tea.

Teapot: A vessel used for brewing and serving tea, which can come in various sizes, shapes, and materials.

Teacup: A small cup used for drinking tea, which can come in various sizes, shapes, and materials.

Index

Introduction:

What is Diabetes?

How Does Tea Affect Blood Sugar Levels?

Benefits of Tea for Diabetes

Tea Types and Varieties

How to Brew Tea

Tips for Enhancing Flavor

Tea Recipes:

Classic Black Tea

Earl Grey Tea

Chai Tea

Green Tea

Matcha Tea

Sencha Tea

Genmaicha Tea

Silver Needle Tea

White Peony Tea

Jasmine Silver Needle Tea

White Tea Lemonade

Chamomile Tea

Ginger Tea

Turmeric Tea

Rooibos Tea

Hibiscus Tea

Peach Tea

Apple Cinnamon Tea

Blueberry Tea

Classic Iced Tea

Green Tea Mint Iced Tea

Mango Iced Tea

Lemon Ginger Iced Tea

Conclusion

Appendix:

Glossary of Tea Terms

Sources and Further Reading

This index covers the different tea types, brewing methods, flavor enhancements, and iced tea options included in the book. Additionally, it includes an introduction to diabetes and tea, as well as a conclusion to wrap up the book. The appendix provides a glossary of tea terms for readers who may not be familiar with certain tea-related terminology and a list of sources for further reading on diabetes and tea.

PLEASE DON'T PLAY WITH YOUR HEALTH.